DEDICATION

This book is dedicated to my mentor and lifelong friend Sandhya. She introduced me to the practice of yoga and I have not looked back since then.

Yoga really gives you that inner peace that so many of us are seeking.

TABLE OF CONTENTS

Yoga Weight Loss: A Complete Guide on Yoga for Beginners

Includes Yoga Poses and Tips on Practicing Yoga

By: Rajesh Aswani

9781632874665

PUBLISHERS NOTES

Disclaimer – Speedy Publishing, LLC

This publication is intended to provide helpful and informative material. It is not intended to diagnose, treat, cure, or prevent any health problem or condition, nor is intended to replace the advice of a physician. No action should be taken solely on the contents of this book. Always consult your physician or qualified health-care professional on any matters regarding your health and before adopting any suggestions in this book or drawing inferences from it.

The author and publisher specifically disclaim all responsibility for any liability, loss or risk, personal or otherwise, which is incurred as a consequence, directly or indirectly, from the use or application of any contents of this book.

Any and all product names referenced within this book are the trademarks of their respective owners. None of these owners have sponsored, authorized, endorsed, or approved this book.

Always read all information provided by the manufacturers' product labels before using their products. The author and publisher are not responsible for claims made by manufacturers.

This book was originally printed before 2014. This is an adapted reprint by Speedy Publishing, LLC with newly updated content designed to help readers with much more accurate and timely information and data.

Speedy Publishing, LLC

40 E Main Street,

Newark

Delaware

19711

Contact Us: 1-888-248-4521

Website: http://www.speedypublishing.com

REPRINTED Paperback Edition: ISBN: 9781632874665

Manufactured in the United States of America

CHAPTER 1- YOGA AN INTRODUCTION

Out of the many things that India is known for in her contribution to the world, 'Yoga' is perhaps one of the most important and popular exports. From the ancient times, the ascetics, the 'rishis' and the 'munis' of India have been practicing this form of art and science and deriving the benefits of enlightenment that accompany yoga.

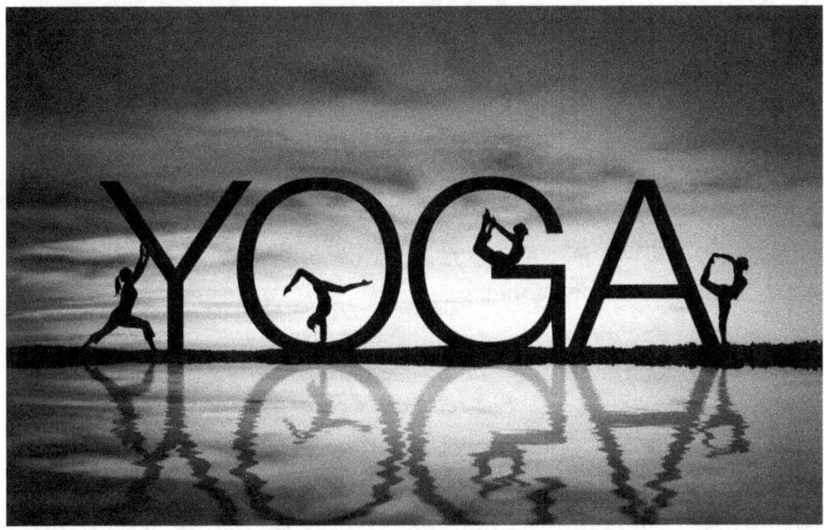

What Is Yoga and Why Is It Important in Today's World?

The importance of yoga in today's world has a lot of definitions floating around; however, if we go back to the roots of the word, we find that the term 'Yoga' has its origins in Sanskrit. It means to unite - Yoga helps the body to unite with the other vital metaphysical aspects of the mind and spirit. It is also often defined as a lifestyle which aims to have a healthy mind within a healthy body.

Yoga Weight Loss

Most simply defined, yoga is a set of poses or 'asanas' , coupled with breathing techniques, which help impart strength and flexibility to the body while helping to balance the mind and its' thinking. Unlike other physical forms of exercises, like the aerobics, by practicing yoga, one can not only achieve physical health, but also mental and spiritual well-being.

The aim of yoga is to promote overall well-being of the body. And though, it is found beneficial for a variety of conditions, it is not considered a therapy for specific illness. Unlike other forms of exercises, yoga has a more holistic approach to teach the people the right way to lead their lives disease free and stress free.

In today's world, all of us suffer from stress and a perpetual anxiety to perform well, leading to a plethora of diseases that we expose ourselves to. Yoga aims to calm and compose our minds and help us focus clearly on what really matters - good health and the happiness that accompanies it!

Benefits of Yoga

Mental Health

Let us first begin with the benefits of Yoga on mental health. After all, good mental health is of paramount importance for being healthy physically as well. As advised above, breathing technique forms an integral part of Yoga. Do I hear you asking 'how?'It really is very basic - by breathing deep and right, something that you would be doing when you practice Yoga, you are inhaling more oxygen and allowing the cells of your body to have access to that oxygen for a longer period of time.

A common practice in yoga is to breathe only from one nostril at a time, while holding the other one closed with the tip of your finger. Medical research has shown that this boosts increased activity of the opposite side of the brain, leading to better cognitive performance and tasks associated with the other side of the brain. Regular yoga practice helps children with attention deficit disorder and people suffering from anxiety, depression and mood swings. It also helps keep the mind calm and reduce stress and thereby increase the general well-being of the person.

Strength

Ever wondered, why so many of us, after a hard day's work, come and plonk ourselves, on our home sofas, with very little energy to even fetch a glass of water for ourselves. This is caused by lack of inner strength. Certain asanas of the yoga help generate inner strength. Inner strength is essential in doing day to day activities and in preventing you from injuries. This is especially useful, as we grow old and need more energy and strength to do the same activity.

Flexibility

The popular notion that you need to be flexible in order to do yoga is incorrect; it is really the other way round - you should do yoga so that you can be more flexible. If you have a flexible body, you find it easy to do tasks. A lot of poses in Yoga concentrate on stretching and improving your flexibility.

With yoga, not only the muscles of the body, but also the softer tissues of your body are worked out, resulting in less build-up of the lactic acid, which is responsible for stiffness in various parts of the body. Yoga increases a range of motions of the less used inner muscles and helps in lubrication of joints. The result is a more flexible body, able to perform tasks easily!

Cardiovascular

Yoga has a lot of positive effects on the cardiovascular system of our body. A healthy cardiovascular system is responsible for preventing heart attacks, strokes and hypertension. Heart disease is a problem which has roots in an improper lifestyle, faulty diet and negative thinking. Our thoughts, emotions and feelings affect our body and negative emotions/thoughts send a series of complex and unhealthy chemical processes throughout the body, giving alarms that something is amiss. Yoga tends to control these by bringing in fresh life-giving oxygen. The anti-oxidant properties of Yoga help in preventing the negative emotions and promote a general well-being in the body.

Joint Pain and Arthritis

The general tendency of people suffering from joint pain, inflammation and stiffness is to avoid exercise. Yoga helps prevent advancement of this malady by toning the muscles and loosening the joints. When a person suffering from joint pain practices yoga, the gentle stretching and strengthening movements of the various Yogic poses, improves the blood flow to the muscles and tissues supporting the joints, thereby making it more comfortable to move.

Respiratory Problems

Practice of certain asanas of Yoga has helped check chronic cases of Asthma and other respiratory problems. When the nasal passages get inflamed, they start producing mucous in excess making it difficult to breathe and often have common symptoms like coughing, wheezing etc. Respiratory problems could also be caused by multiple factors like allergy, exercise, weather change etc. By practicing yoga, the lungs capacities increase and so does stamina and stress on air passages is reduced.

Back pain• Yoga has helped innumerable cases of back ache. Back ache is caused due to stress and tension in the muscles supporting the spinal cord. Back ache may be caused due to improper postures mild injuries, which have been left untreated etc. Yoga has seemed to help cases of back pain by enhancing flexibility and strengthening the muscle groups supporting the spine, helping the body to maintain an upright posture. It eases the back pain by increase in blood circulation and getting healing nutrients to the injured muscles. Apart from healing injured muscles, it also prevents further injuries by strengthening the muscles.

Memory Improvement

"Memory is the measure of ability to reproduce the knowledge that is known", says Yogacharya Vishwas.

"Memory is holding on to that which has been known."- The Hindu Texts.

Yoga helps in retaining information better and for a longer period of time due to its focus on concentration and meditation. By breathing right, concentrating and meditating, more blood flows to the brain, making it supple and ready to accept more information and reproduce that information when required.

Obesity

Obesity is when a person weighs more than his normal/ stipulated weight. This may be caused due to faulty eating habits, stress related eating, imbalances in the digestive and endocrine system or even something as basic as less physical exercise. Yoga helps obesity by inhaling more oxygen, which helps in breaking down fat cells and increasing your metabolism. Also, it helps remove sluggishness from the digestive and endocrine systems, making them work better.

Anti-Ageing

Regular practice of yoga has anti ageing effects. Yoga revitalizes the mind and makes the approach towards life positive and stress free. Apart from this, a person practicing yoga regularly is more flexible, fit and mentally agile. Overall happiness and positive attitude towards life reflects on the face, leaving it glowing and reverses the ageing effect internally.

The importance of yoga in today's world has a whole lot of other everyday benefits such as sound and deep sleep, high energy levels etc. However, the key to deriving these benefits is to be consistent with Yogic practices and do it under the supervision of a well-trained yoga teacher.

Chapter 2- What You Need To Practice Yoga

Yoga Equipment

There are many items available for those who practice yoga. None of them are truly required, but there are many that would be especially helpful.

You may have even seen a number of them in videos, on television, or in your local store. Perhaps you didn't even realize they were used for yoga.

For many years yoga equipment was hard to find and somewhat expensive. Now it's very prevalent and the prices on most equipment are very affordable.

The problem is, the prevalence of equipment makes it hard to decide what you need and what you don't. You don't need everything, no matter what the salesperson may try to tell you.

We're going to look at some of the most popular types of yoga equipment and accessories so you can decide what you need, what you might want, and what you can live without.

If you're just getting started you really need very little, especially if you'll be taking a class. Your class may provide the items you need, but not all will. You'll probably need to bring your own mat at the very least.

The equipment you buy will also largely be a personal choice. You may not need to buy something that someone else would consider essential.

For example, you'll find some people who prefer to sit on a hard floor or on the ground outdoors. Others find it very uncomfortable to sit on a hard surface and may feel pain in their back and tailbone. These people would really need a yoga mat.

I'm going to simply describe each item and let you make your own judgments as to what is right for you. I won't try to tell you what you should and shouldn't buy, but I will tell you what I feel might be helpful.

Yoga Mats

For most people, a yoga mat will be essential. A lot of people won't be able to comfortably sit on the floor without a mat, and this can be very discouraging. You may be fine without one, but it's something you should consider.

The first thing you should look for in a yoga mat is a good floor grip. You're not going to want a mat that will slip around a lot, especially while you're attempting difficult postures.

You'll also want to choose a mat with enough padding to make it comfortable.

You'll find yoga mats in different sizes, thicknesses, and colors, so you'll be able to find one to suit you. If you're going to buy one, you should be sure to find one that you're really happy with.

Yoga Towel

There are special towels that are made for yoga. You may find super-absorbent towels that will be quite helpful if you sweat a lot, and you may even find these in "chakra colors" which you can use in various situations.

You may also buy a skidless towel that you can use on your mat to help absorb sweat. This may be especially important if you practice Bikram yoga.

Yoga Bags

If you buy a lot of yoga accessories you may want to buy a special bag to carry them. They look like duffel bags, and are often made of nylon.

Yoga Straps

If you have trouble holding your poses you might wish to buy yoga straps. They can help you hold those difficult poses longer.

Yoga Sandbags and Bolsters

Sandbags and bolsters can help you keep your balance and support you through your poses. They come in many colors, and you may be able to match your outfit, mat, and other accessories.

Yoga Meditation Seating

Meditation seating comes in a variety of different types. You can buy special cushions, benches, and pillows for various poses, and they make it very comfortable for meditating for longer periods of time.

Yoga Balls

For around $25 you can buy a yoga ball. They help you learn balance, build your strength, tone your muscles, and make it comfortable for people with injuries to exercise.

These balls provide extra support as you stretch, and are good for working out the back and hips, and can also be used during pregnancy.

You'll need an air pump if you get one of these. The air will slowly come out of the ball as you use it, causing it to deflate after several uses, so you shouldn't forget to buy a pump to fill it back up.

Yoga Blocks

Yoga blocks are somewhat like mattresses. They have a number of uses, but they are most commonly used for body movement extensions.

Yoga Videos

Many people love to pick up videos they can use at home. They may not have the money for formal classes, or they may feel shy or awkward about attending classes with other people. Perhaps they just don't have a lot of extra time.

Videos are a really good way to get into yoga if you can't take formal yoga classes. You'll be able to get in more practice and feel more comfortable doing some of the poses at home. If you decide later to take formal classes you'll already be a little ahead of some of the others in the class, especially if you start in beginners' classes.

Yoga Music

There are special CDs you can buy that are made to enhance the meditation experience. These can be used for enhancing the tranquility you experience.

There are also CDs that help with your flow, including trance music. You may also find chants and mantras on CD that can help you get into the right frame of mind.

Yoga Clothing

You don't need any special clothing for practicing yoga unless you just want to buy some. Many people like to exercise in full leotards of different types, but a comfortable cotton t-shirt and stretchy leggings that breathe would be just fine.

CHAPTER 3- THE LINK BETWEEN MEDITATION & YOGA

Meditation is an important part of yoga. It deserves its own section, because it has such an important place in your yoga practice.

While yoga often focuses a little more on the physical side with a secondary emphasis on mental health, meditation is more about mental health with a secondary emphasis on physical health.

Even a few minutes of meditation each day can help you reduce stress levels significantly. And lowering your stress levels has the additional positive effect of reducing blood pressure, stabilizing heart and respiration rates, and boosting your immune system.

Meditation uses the standard stages of the mind to cause certain effects at certain times. Let's take a look at these different states.

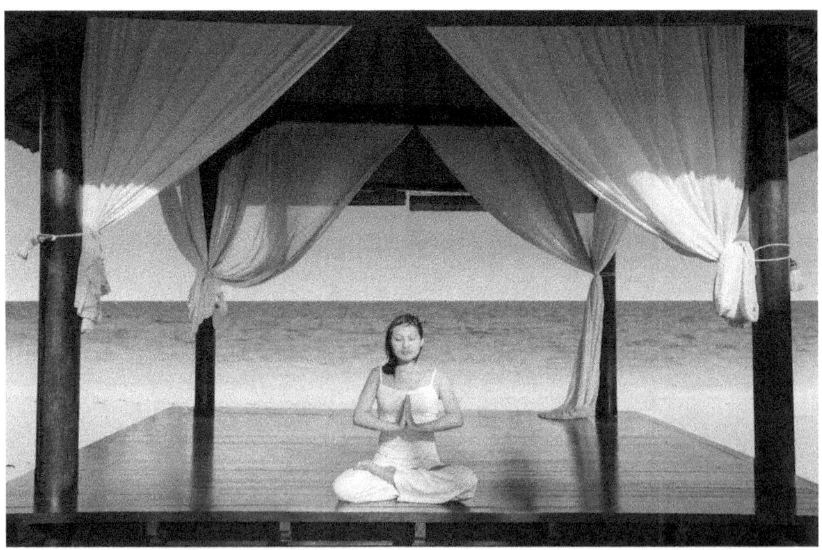

Stage One: The Normal State of Mind

When your mind is in this state you are awake and being stimulated. You react normally, and you are thinking.

During this phase your mind may jump around and wander a lot. You may be performing one task, and you may notice something that reminds you of something else and sends you off on a tangent.

During this phase the mind is very active, but also very distractible. This can cause you a lot of problems if you're driving or working or doing something else that requires quite a lot of concentration.

This is the state of the mind in which stress tends to build up heavily. If your stress gets out of control you may find it very difficult to concentrate and you may start to fall behind on your work or daily tasks.

Stage Two: The Concentration State of Mind

During this phrase, you will enter the first state that carries you toward the state of meditation. Concentration isn't the state of meditation itself, but it is closer to it than the standard waking state of mind.

Concentration can actually be extremely difficult to master. You have to learn to focus on one single thing to the exclusion of everything else.

The mind can easily pull you back into a normal state until you learn how to control it. It may take you days, weeks, months, or even years to perfect this. If your mind is extremely active and you are easily distracted, this may be a difficult for you, but you can do it.

Let's look at an example of how distractions work. You don't have to be distracted by an event happening live around you. Your own mind can actually distract you.

Let's say you're sitting at work and you're concentrating on a complex piece of paperwork. You see the name of a client on a piece of paper, and her name is the same as your sister. This reminds you that you were supposed to call her about a concert the two of you are supposed to attend during the upcoming weekend. Then you start thinking of how much fun the concert will be and what you will wear.

Has something like this happened to you? Something similar has happened to most of us, if not all of us. Our minds have the power to inject thoughts almost spontaneously when we encounter something that triggers it. Sometimes there doesn't even need to be a trigger.

When you practice concentration, your goal is to recognize this and immediately snap back into concentration. When you master concentration, you'll be surprised at how your mind will function better and how much more you will be able to relax!

Stage Three: The Full Meditation State of Mind

In the third stage of the process, your mind will have finally freed itself of any internal or external distractions from stimuli. No distractions will be able to affect you during this stage unless they are very serious or purposeful.

Many people claim they have discovered things about themselves or learned things they believe they never would have learned if they didn't enter meditation.

In meditation you are able to keep your thoughts centered onto one thing. You'll be able to concentrate on a particular thought and make it part of you.

It will take you some time and practice to learn to control the stages of your mind, but you'll be rewarded with better concentration, better problem solving, and a great way to reduce stress.

Stage Four: The Contemplation State of Mind

The final level of meditation is the contemplation level. This is a very difficult level to understand without actually experiencing it for yourself.

During this phase, you will enter a new type of consciousness. You've probably never entered this phase before, so it may be quite surprising the first time.

Instead of focusing on your own issues as most people do, you will instead connect with the world itself. Your own body and mind will be completely secondary to you, and you will finally realize just how small we each are, and how very vast the universe is.

It won't be easy to get to this phase. You may not reach it until you've practiced meditation many times. You were born with the ability to do this, but you have to actually practice it in order to achieve it.

The Purpose of Meditation

Meditation has many benefits. The most important one for many people is reaching enlightenment in the Contemplation phase, but this may not be important to everyone.

Some people only want to use meditation as a way to become more spiritual, or do control stress or panic attacks, or to treat physical pain or illnesses.

You don't have to meditate for the purpose of enlightenment or spirituality if that is of no interest to you. In fact, there are many people who don't even believe in spirituality of any kind but still use meditation as a way to relax and heal their mind and body.

Some executives use meditation as a way to ease their mind the way sleep does. In their busy lives, they may not get as much sleep as they really need, so they can use 5-10 minutes of meditation to refresh their mind when they feel stressed out, tired, distracted, or have trouble concentrating.

Parents often use meditation as a way to calm the stress of daily life so they don't end up angry at their children. This is a great way to stay calm.

Meditation is a very good anger management tool. If you have anger issues, you may use meditation as a way to get the condition under control.

Let's Look At Some of the Major Benefits of Meditation

- ❖ Meditation helps you focus more clearly. You'll be more efficient and you'll get more done in less time.
- ❖ Meditation will help you reduce your stress levels.
- ❖ Meditation will help you learn to be more sympathetic to other people, and more understanding.
- ❖ Mediation will help you become a kinder, more compassionate person.
- ❖ Meditation helps you communicate with others on a better, more effective level.

- ❖ Meditation can improve blood pressure, heart rate, and respiration, and even assist in managing heart disease.
- ❖ Meditation can help boost your immune system by lowering your stress levels.
- ❖ Meditation can help boost your memory and concentration through boosting oxygen levels.
- ❖ Meditation can help your mind achieve the kind of clarity you never thought you could experience.

These are just a few of the different benefits you may achieve through meditation.

There are so many additional benefits that are experienced by different people it would be very difficult to list them all here!

CHAPTER 4- YOGA FOR WEIGHT LOSS

In today's society, obesity is a cause for concern with even children that are overweight. Apart from eating healthy, it is worth looking at the importance of yoga and weight loss.

Weight gain is not only about the number of calories taken in. There are other underlying causes in the body that will result to weight gain if they become unbalanced. The use of yoga posture can be very helpful in redressing this balance hence helping the body to burn fat more effectively resulting in healthy weight loss.

Some vital functions of the body that can be improved by yoga and help promote weight loss:

The Liver

The liver is the body's own detoxifying machine. A healthy liver works effectively to cleanse the blood of bad fat and helps the blood make use the good fat. Certain yoga postures help increase the functions of the liver. A healthy liver will remove bad fat effectively. Yoga postures like cobra pose and bow pose can be used.

The Thyroid Gland

Yoga and weight loss program can also involve poses that stimulate the thyroid gland. The hormone that governs the body's metabolism is in the thyroid. How high or low a body's metabolism is depends on how active the thyroid is. Most weight gain issues are due to hypothyroidism meaning low thyroid activity. Activating the thyroid function by using postures like fish pose and shoulder stand will help greatly towards weight loss.

The Nervous System

It is not necessary to attend a hot yoga class to generate body heat. Internal heat is created in the body using nerve tension heat and length. This internal heat can burn deep and low seated fat. This can be achieved using the lunge and the seated forward bend.

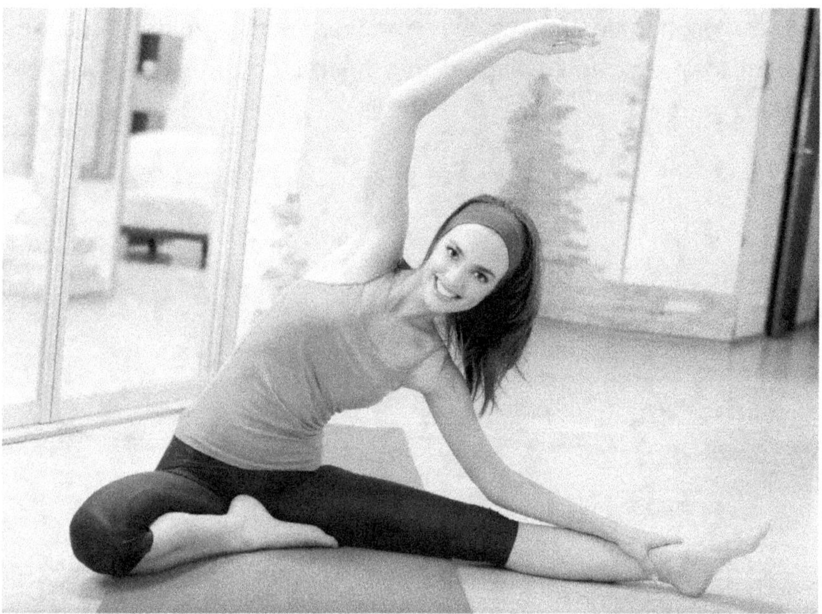

Heart Rate

It is very common to see people jogging to get their heart rate up in the quest to lose weight. This has been proven to stress the nervous system. Since a perfectly working nervous system is needed to aid in the yoga and weight loss program, any activity that adds stress to the nervous system should be avoided. It is better in the case of loss weight to use activities that raises the heart rate for a short period and then back down. This can be easily done using yoga.

Body Movements

Yoga Weight Loss

Yoga exercises that work to lengthen and shorten the muscles will aid in weight loss. Muscles use fat as fuel and will continue to do so even while in rest position. Strength exercises such as arm balancing will work well as they work all body muscles at once. Recommended yoga postures include crane and scale pose.

In Ayurveda, it is said that the issue is not to lose weight but to avoid weight gain. As we will discover in this guide, Yoga and weight loss programs will lead to a healthy, slimmer and younger looking you!

CHAPTER 5- THE EVOLUTION OF YOGA

Whether you are a yoga fan or are just now discovering the art, knowledge of the history of yoga can help you appreciate its origin, understand it as a life transforming facet and effectively incorporate it into your life to shed those extra pounds and experience what yoga has to offer.

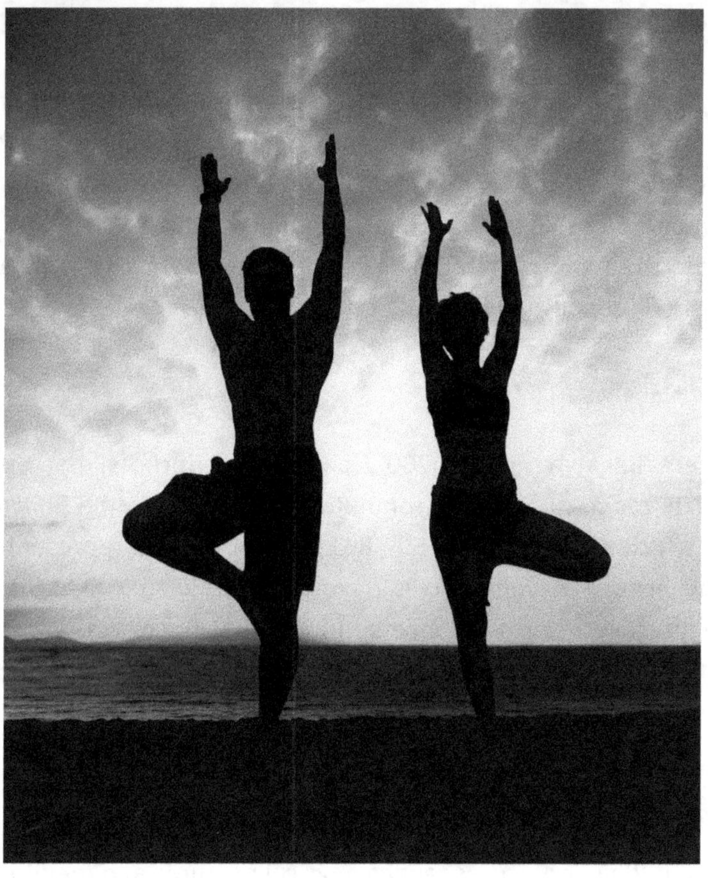

So we must start at the beginning. Yoga is believed to be as old as civilization. Scholars have traced the origin of yoga to Stone Age Shamanism. Like yoga, Shamanism's major aim was to improve the condition of human life, heal community members and act as a spiritual mediator.

The earliest archaeological evidence depicting the history of Yoga dates back to 3000 B.C. It is found in stone seals featuring yoga poses. More effectively, yoga history is divided into four periods which clearly detail its evolution into the modern yoga. These include:

Vedic

This period is represented by the Vedas; the sacred scripture of Hinduism. The Vedas have evidence of the oldest Yogic teachings called Vedic Yoga or Archaic Yoga. Vedic Yoga involved rituals and ceremonies designed to connect people to the spirit world and surpass the mind's limitations. Vedic yogis; also called rishis were consulted for spiritual illumination.

Pre-Classical

This era began with the 200 Upanishad scriptures that related ultimate reality to the transcendental self. However, the Bhagavad-Gita, which was created in 500 B.C., is a more vivid representation of the history of yoga and is devoted entirely to Yoga. The Gita brought together three facets: Bhakti (loving devotion), Jnana (contemplation or knowledge) and Karma (selfless actions). By so doing, it united Bhakti, Jnana and Karma yoga.

It was also during the pre-classical period that yoga found its way into Buddhism, with Lord Buddha being the first Buddhist to study yoga. Buddhist scriptures taught physical postures and meditation.

Classical

Classical yoga is marked by the creation of Yoga Sutras by Patanjali. The 195 maxims expound on Raja Yoga using Patanjali's Eightfold path of yoga or the Eight Limbs of Classical Yoga which are: Yama (ethical values) Niyama (observing purity, tolerance and study) Asanas (physical exercise) Pranayama (controlled breathing) Pratyahara (withdrawing to prepare for meditation) Dharana (concentration) Dhyana (meditation)Samadhi (ecstasy)

Post Classical

This is the most modern era marked by an abundance of yoga literature and widened yoga practice. Post-classical yoga differs from previous yoga practices in that it teaches one to accept reality and live in the moment rather, than get liberated from reality.

Yoga found its way into the West in the early 19th century. It was first studied as Eastern Philosophy before becoming popular among vegetarians and health conscious people in the 1930s. By 1960s several Indian yogis had popularized yoga such as Maharishi Mahesh who taught Transcendental Meditation and Sivananda who popularized the now widely used principles of yoga, which include:

Savasana (proper relaxation) Asanas (physical exercise) Pranayama (proper breathing) Dhyana (meditation and positive thinking) Proper diet

Today, yoga has crossed geographical and spiritual boundaries and is practiced globally as a means for health and wellness.

CHAPTER 6- WEIGHT LOSS WITH YOGA- THE GUIDELINES

According to the yogic, man's problem is not being awakened enough to know the inner self.

In yoga, breathing is considered the source of life and breathing exercises and postures are used to connect with the spirit. For a beginner wishing to take on yoga, some guidelines when beginning yoga are in order to help appreciate the experience more. The main issues are where, when, what and how to practice yoga

Where Is the Best Place to Practice?

Yoga can be practiced at home on in a yoga class. It can be practiced indoors as well as outdoor. For indoor sessions, select a particular area and turn off any noise source. If warmth is needed, a yoga mat or any exercise mat can be used. When practicing outside, shaded areas are better.

When Is It Recommended To Practice?

The first thing is to choose a time when there will be no disturbance or distraction. Also there is no need to rush so choose the right time. The experience will be better and effective if the stomach is empty so wait at least two hours after meals. The postures also called asana will be best taken when the body is relatively flexible. Choose the right time of the day during which your body is most flexible. Most guidelines when beginning yoga will suggest sessions of at least ten minutes of posture. If meditation is to be added, this could be increased to about twenty minutes or more.

How Is the Practice Done?

Yoga is practiced on bare feet. Bare feet not only help in taking the right posture but also help prevent slipping. Wear clothing that is loose and comfortable enough to allow the different postures to be taken.

What Postures (Asana) To Take?

Yoga is not about force and any exercise that creates tension in the body should be abandoned. Even before you beginning taking postures, it is important to understand your own body and how it can go. Yoga is not done for competition and patience and effort will pay off.

Other Guidelines When Beginning Yoga

1. Always begin each session with a warm-up. Use exercises the stretch the spine and legs.
2. Understand inhalation and exhalation procedures. Inhalations are associated with expanding movements and exhalation with contracting movements.
3. Sequencing is the change from one pose to another. This helps to balance the workout session.
4. Understand the different uses of the various poses.
5. Always breathe through the nose.
6. Start with simple postures and move up as you get more comfortable.
7. Always avoid injury by not forcing the body into a particular posture.
8. Always end the session by relaxing the body.

Like in all exercises, starting simple and getting complex later will yield more benefit. With yoga, constant practice session is the key to getting better. Postures are repeated three times but instead of trying to do a posture thrice, try to get it right even once. Hopefully these guidelines when beginning yoga classes will prove useful to those considering yoga.

CHAPTER 7- HOW TO AVOID THE TYPICAL MISTAKES

Uncertainties are normal whenever you start on something new and these uncertainties could lead to negative first impressions, thus resulting to backing out and not wanting to try the same activity again. The same goes with yoga. Yoga exercises can provide you with lots of benefits, both physical and spiritual and missing out on its important elements can result to negative results. Avoiding yoga beginner's mistakes is of utmost importance and 3 of these common mistakes include the following:

Not Knowing What You Want From the Practice

You may not be aware of the fact that there are various styles and forms of yoga and these have their own different attractions. Before enrolling in a yoga class, it is necessary to determine first what attracted you to yoga and from there; you can start investigating the different styles that will cater to your attraction. You can set goals and these goals can be mental, physical or spiritual. Once you have set your goal, you can now discuss this with your yoga instructor before you begin with the classes. Your instructor will be able to discuss with you your goals and give you advice on how you can easily achieve it. However, make sure that you have a set timeframe for these goals to make it more measureable.

Jumping in Feet First

Once they have decided to attend a yoga class, some people tend to head on and jump to a 12 month class. Take note that these classes normally require an upfront payment and it progresses from one level and so on as the week progresses. Although learning yoga is fantastic, you should not opt for a 12 month class, as you are not yet sure if the class you opted for is ideal for you. The best thing that you can do is to join beginner yoga classes first. Once you have attended these classes, you can easily determine the type of yoga that you want for yourself and your goal.

As these classes were designed to give students a broader understanding on the different types of yoga, the levels of students also vary and the instructors are normally strict. However, this is beneficial for you because as mentioned, it can help you determine the type of yoga that will be most suitable for you without involving any huge financial outlay. You will not be required to attend every class as well, so you will not fall behind when you miss a class, unlike in longer courses of yoga.

Choosing the Wrong Instructor

Yoga instructors should have been an apprentice of a skilled guru for several years before being able to teach simple yoga techniques. However, there are yoga instructors who just went through a 3-day course and this will definitely make a huge difference. Proper yoga techniques can be achieved depending on the level of abilities and skills of the instructor that is why it is necessary to find the right instructor for your yoga class. Although unqualified yoga instructors are not necessarily terrible, qualified instructors are still your best option.

Avoiding yoga beginner's mistakes can help you succeed in learning yoga techniques and in achieving your goals. If you can avoid the common mistakes mentioned above, it would be a lot easier for you to learn this practice and be able to reap its benefits without wasting your time and effort.

CHAPTER 8- YOGA POSTURES: ASANAS

Yoga is carried out by making postures known as asanas. These postures ensure that the person doing yoga is relaxed for a specific duration. In the modern age, there are many postures that are made to exercise both the body and mind.

Asanas: Yoga Postures—the Fundamental Yoga Poses Types - basically, there are four types of yoga postures with many sub-postures. These four postures are standing yoga poses, sitting yoga poses, yoga poses while lying down on back and yoga poses while lying down on the stomach.

Standing Yoga Poses

These are yoga poses that are done when one is standing. Under this category of yoga postures, there are various different postures that can be made such as: standing sideways while bending one arm; bending sideways while using both arms; standing on a spinal twist; bending forward while standing; bending backwards while standing; making a triangle pose; making a warrior pose; bending forward with the feet apart; making a tree pose; making a chair pose; bending forward while standing on one leg.

Sitting Yoga Poses

These are yoga poses that are done when one is sitting. Under this category of yoga postures, there are various different postures that can be made such as: making and inclined plane posture; sitting with a half spinal twist posture; sitting with a butterfly posture; making a cat stretch; making a child posture; making a mill churning posture; making a bow pose; making a cobra pose.

Yoga Poses While Lying On the Back

Yoga Weight Loss

These are yoga poses that are done when one is lying on the back. Under this category of yoga postures, there are various different postures that can be made such as: superman pose; fish pose; locust pose; bridge pose; boat pose.

Yoga Poses While Lying On the Stomach

These are yoga poses that are done when one is lying on the stomach. Under this category of yoga postures, there are various different postures that can be made such as: shoulder stand; wind-relieving pose; plow pose; lying-down body twist; corpse pose; lying-down on sides.

Asanas: Yoga Postures—the Fundamental Yoga Poses Practices

Whenever carrying out asanas, there are practices that are observed. For instance, one should perform the positions on an empty stomach. This is in order to avoid constipation. When making the postures, force, or else pressure, must not be applied. The body should be stable and trembling completely avoided. The head in particular, as well as other body parts, such as the heels, must be lowered slowly to avoid any physical injury. Whenever the postures are being made, breathing should be well controlled.

Advantages of Yoga

There are many advantages that come along with taking up yoga. These include: Improving flexibility; improving balance; improving strength; reducing anxiety and stress; reducing lower back pain symptoms; reducing hypertension; shortening labor; improving fitness/physical health; reducing sleep disorders; decreasing fatigue while increasing energy.

With such benefits to the health, mentality, and fitness, yoga is surely a practice that all should undertake, whether young or elderly.

CHAPTER 9- HOW TO MODIFY THE DIET

Ideally, it is always a good idea that you conduct yoga practice without eating anything too close prior to beginning. But as it is not possible all the time because of personal and professional commitments, you need to be very careful of what you are eating.

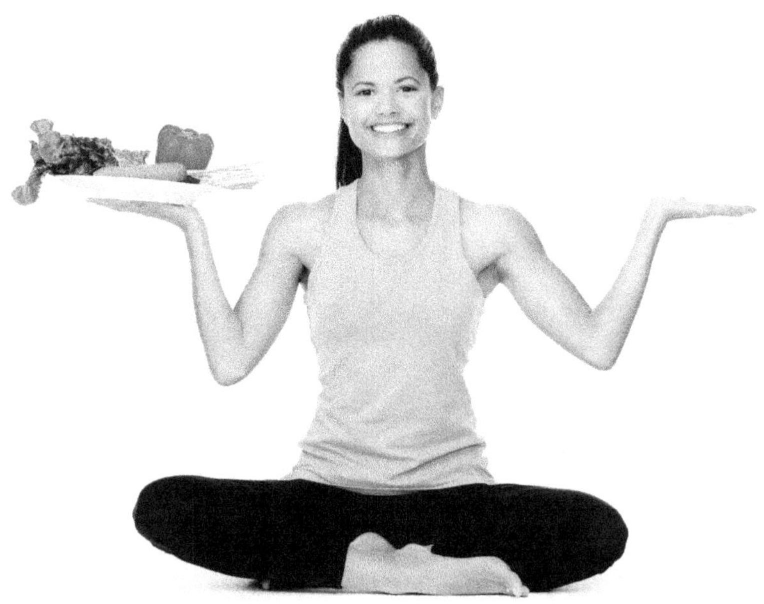

Timing

Timing is quite pivotal. If you are interested in a light meal before going for yoga practice, it is advisable that you take it one to two hours beforehand. When you follow this strategy, it will give your digestive system quite a bit of time to settle down. This will ensure that you are going to feel at ease during class.

For people interested in heavier meal, the time frame should be in the vicinity of four to five hours.

Fruits and Vegetables

Your first preference should be fruits and vegetables. One of the most important things about fruits and vegetables is that you are not going to have any digestive issues and in a matter of hour, you will get a feeling of empty stomach. In addition, inclusion of fruits and vegetables in your diet is advantageous for your overall health.

Heavy Foods

Make sure that you stay away from heavy foods. Before yoga class, you should not eat meats, pasta and processed grains. After eating these foods, you are going to feel lethargic, which is not ideal when you are all set to give your all in your yoga workout.

Spicy Foods

Similar to heavy foods, you should also stay away from spicy foods. Because of the fact that spicy foods can easily lead to heartburn, you should not take these foods before starting the yoga practice.

Talking about yoga, not only it has an impact on the outside portion of your body but also inside portion and therefore you can pretty much imagine how it is going to be when you fill your stomach with spicy foods.

Yoghurt

Before going for yoga practice, it is always a good thing to try yogurt. Taking yoghurt half an hour before the yoga class is not only going to be good for your digestion but also the strengthening of your heart.

Final Diet Tips

No two individuals are same and therefore you will find that there is going to be variation in terms of diet as well. It's not easy figuring out an ideal time for eating before yoga. But as the time passes by and you get to know about your body, more notably, your digestive system, you will be able to plan out things in a much better manner.

Individuals with low blood sugar need to eat something fifty minutes before yoga practice. When it comes to yoga practice, use of nuts is recommended. Almonds, pecans and walnuts contain essential iron and vitamins, good for your health. For healthy intestinal tract, pecans are one of the best options. There are lots of poses in yoga that are going to have a positive impact on the intestines. To get the best out of this, you need to take pecans and walnuts on a regular basis.

CHAPTER 10- BEST YOGA POSES FOR WEIGHT LOSS

The most effective yoga poses for weight loss can actually make you lose weight just like employing other high impact exercises. Yoga is known for being a stress-relieving method, but it has also been proven by many people to be an effective weight loss remedy. Yoga started as a means of meditation from ancient civilization and was very popular in Hinduism.

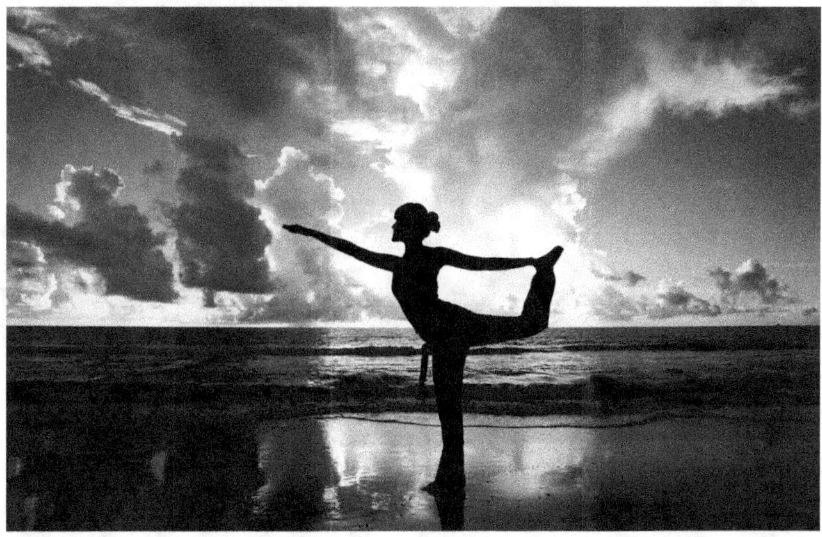

Yoga is beneficial for the overall health not only just the physical aspect of people. Among the benefits of which include better equilibrium, increased reaction time, improved energy levels, enhanced sleep, improved memory and concentration, reduced depression and anxiety and many others.

For people who want to lose weight, it has been proven that yoga is also effective for the normalization of weight. The most effective yoga poses for weight loss actually helps you maintain a desirable weight because they tend to increase the metabolism while these poses are being employed. Also, it improves the overall circulation to effectively utilize glucose and fats for energy production instead of being stored as fats.

Not only do they increase burning of fats, they also tone major muscle groups for a leaner body. So to help you maintain a normal weight, the following are the most effective yoga poses for weight loss that you can do at home:

Crescent

This yoga pose tones firms the thighs, hips and abs. Stand with your feet together and your arms at your sides. Breathe in deeply and raise your arms overhead in a straight manner. Slowly exhale and bend your knees forward while lowering your hands to the floor. Inhale and exhale while assuming a lunge position and bring your arms overhead again.

Willow

This position helps you tone your legs, arms and behind. Stand with your feet together and your arms at your sides. Lift your legs and place the sole of your right foot against the inner left thigh ensuring your knees are turned to the side. Position your arms in front of your chest with palms facing each other. Extend your arms up towards the ceiling. Bend torso to your right. Repeat for 5 times after which do it on your other side.

Twisted Chair Pose

This is one of the most effective yoga poses for weight loss because it improves the circulation and calorie burning by using each and every major and minor muscle groups in your body. Stand with your feet together. Bend at your knees and assume a position as if you are sitting on a chair far behind your back. Place your palms facing each other in front of your chest. Rotate and bring your left elbow to your right knee. Hold the position for 30 seconds and release. Repeat on the other side.

Locust Pose

This is another one of the most effective yoga poses for weight loss as it strengthens your lower back and legs. It also boosts your energy levels to make you feel an increased feeling of well-being. Lie on your abdomen with arms on your side facing the ceiling. Lift your head, arms, legs and body off the floor as if the only ones in contact with the floor is your stomach. Hold the position as high as possible and feel your muscles contract. Release after 30 seconds and repeat three to five times.

Bow Pose

This is similar to the locust position only that your arms reach for your legs so you are doing a more difficult pose. First, perform the locust position. Bend your knees up ward so your arms can grab your ankles. Make your position as relaxed as possible to prevent muscle strain. Hold the position for 30 seconds and repeat three times.

You can actually do more poses, but remember not to miss these out because they are just some of the most effective yoga poses for weight loss.

CONCLUSION

As we have learnt throughout this guide, Yoga is more than just stretching; it is a spiritual experience as well as a physical one mastering exercises and postures as well as your breathing. Yoga is considered by some to be an alternative for medicine. It has a lot of benefits not only to the physical but also to the mental state of a person. So to conclude this beginner's guide we will recap what we have just covered

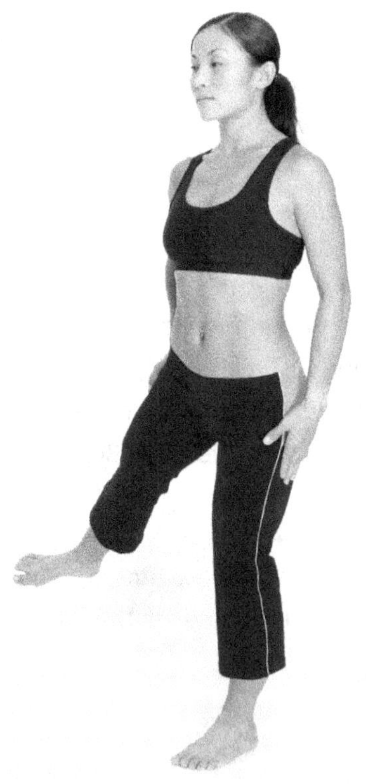

Where Did Yoga Originate?

Yoga is believed to have been in existence since thousands of years ago even before the ancient people learned the writing system. It originated in India where its name was derived from the Sanskrit word yui which roughly translate to English as unite. Experts believe that the practice was named this way because it unites the body, the mind and the soul into one to create a holistic effect. Over the years, more and more techniques are created to make a better yoga experience for people who want to improve their overall health condition.

What Are The Benefits Of Yoga?

The Physical Aspect

Some people started practicing yoga because they wanted to become more flexible. The practice involves different poses where muscles have to be stretched. This is very useful for people who have arthritis and those who are in their old age. As the body ages, the bones become more rigid and the muscles become weak. With yoga, even elderly people can move like they are 20 years younger.

Yoga poses are specially designed to improve the core strength of the body. As people continually practice the positions, the muscles are becoming more and more toned. After doing yoga for several weeks, you will realize that your stamina has improved and you will feel stronger.

With yoga's focus on poses, posture will be dramatically enhanced. A lot of medical conditions are brought about by poor posture which include spinal cord problems, chronic fatigue syndrome and back pain. Good posture, on the other hand, will improve the circulation of blood in the body and will result to a healthier and more alert mind.

The Mental Aspect

Yoga focuses more on breathing than perfecting the poses especially for beginner classes. Proper breathing will help clear the mind and reduce stress. With effective meditation techniques, people will be able to create more sound decisions and these will prevent them from acting out of whim.

Practicing yoga will prove to be essential in fighting depression and increasing concentration. When a person is depressed, a lot of things fill the mind and this can lead to several accidents involving poor concentration. This can directly affect work and daily routines.

How Does One Get Started With Yoga?

Although it is perfectly fine to practice yoga at home with instructional videos, it is still recommended for beginners to take basic lessons. Learning the proper way of breathing and the proper way of doing basic poses will be helpful to maximize the health benefits. Everyone should have all the necessary items which include yoga mats, straps and proper attire. Knowing the basic order will also help beginners prepare for the sessions. Warm-up poses are done during the first few minutes followed by the poses in their respective order - standing, sitting, twists, supine and prone. Finishing poses are done at the last part of the session which aims to cool down the body.

Yoga is great for everyone. Don't procrastinate and start yoga today to reap the benefits

ABOUT THE AUTHOR

Rajesh Aswani never started practicing yoga until he was introduced to it by his friend Sandyha. He was a skeptic but he was open to trying it and then making the decision as to whether or not it was the right move to make.

He had only positive benefits from his experience and started to spread the word on his experience supported by facts about the real benefits of yoga. He encourages his readers to do same, to try yoga and decide for themselves if it is for them.